Table of Contents

Introduction

Chapter 1:-Understanding Emotional Eating

Chapter 2:-The Mind-Body Connection

Chapter 3:-Identifying Your Emotional Triggers

Chapter 4:-Overcoming Mindset Barriers

B. Strategies to change limiting beliefs
C. Cultivating a growth mindset

Chapter 5:-Mindful Eating

A. Introduction to mindful eating
B. Mindful eating techniques and practices
C. Benefits of mindful eating

Chapter 6:-Building a Support System

A. The importance of a support system
B. Finding support in your community
C. Online resources and communities

Chapter 7:-Creating a Sustainable Weight Loss Plan

A. Setting realistic goals
B. Designing a personalized weight loss plan
C. Incorporating long-term strategies

Chapter 8:-Coping with Setbacks

A. How to handle relapses and setbacks
B. Developing resilience and self-compassion

Conclusion
   A. Summarizing key takeaways
   B. Encouragement for the journey ahead

Introduction

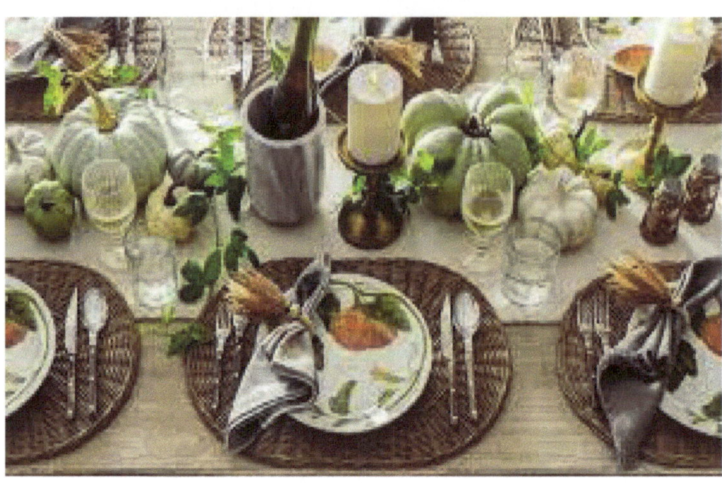

A. The Link Between Emotions and Eating

Emotions are powerful drivers of our behavior. They can dictate our choices, actions, and even the food we consume. Whether it's the joy of celebration, the comfort of solace, or the stress of a long day, our emotions often find expression through what we eat. This connection between our emotional state and eating habits is something most of us can relate to. It's not just about sustenance; it's about seeking solace, finding joy, or numbing pain in the foods we consume.

B. **The Importance of Addressing Mindset Barriers**

When it comes to weight loss and overall well-being, it's not just about counting calories or hitting the gym. Your mindset plays a pivotal role in determining your success. The way you think about food, your body, and your ability to make lasting changes profoundly influences your journey to a healthier you. Mindset barriers can often be the invisible roadblocks that hinder progress. They can be rooted in self-doubt, limiting beliefs, or past experiences. Addressing these mindset barriers is the key to unlocking your full potential and achieving sustainable weight loss.

In this ebook, we will delve into the intricate relationship between emotions and eating. We will explore the emotions that drive us to the kitchen, the pantry, or the drive-thru, and we'll equip you with the knowledge and tools to navigate these emotional waters. Furthermore, we will dissect the powerful role that mindset plays in your quest for weight loss. It's not just about what you eat, but how you think about what you eat that can make all the difference.

Join us on this journey as we uncover the complexities of emotional eating and help you break free from the mindset barriers that have held you back. It's time to reclaim control over your relationship with food, your emotions, and ultimately, your health.

Chapter 1: Understanding Emotional Eating

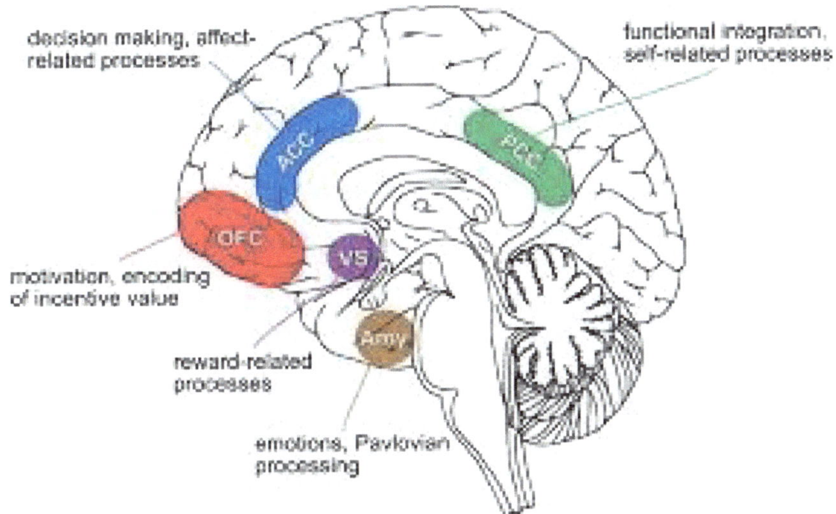

A. What is Emotional Eating?

Emotional eating is a term that encapsulates a behavior many of us are familiar with, yet may not fully comprehend. Simply put, it refers to the act of consuming food not for the purpose of nourishment or physical hunger but in response to emotional triggers. These emotional triggers can include a wide range of feelings, such as stress, sadness, boredom, loneliness, anxiety, or even happiness. Emotional eating is when we turn to food as a coping mechanism, a source of comfort, or as a way to suppress or deal with our emotions.

Have you ever found yourself reaching for a tub of ice cream after a tough day at work, or devouring a bag of chips while feeling stressed? These are classic examples of emotional eating. It's important to recognize that emotional eating is a common behavior, and it doesn't make you weak or undisciplined. Instead, it highlights the powerful connection between your emotions and your food choices.

B. **The Emotional Triggers Behind It**

Understanding emotional eating goes beyond recognizing the behavior itself. It's essential to delve into the emotional triggers that lead to it. Emotional triggers are the specific emotions or situations that prompt you to seek solace or distraction in food. These triggers can be diverse and may vary from person to person. Some individuals may turn to food when they're feeling overwhelmed by stress, while others may eat to celebrate moments of happiness. Identifying your personal emotional triggers is a crucial step in addressing emotional eating, as it allows you to develop strategies to manage these emotions without turning to food.

C. **The Consequences of Emotional Eating**

While emotional eating may offer temporary relief from emotional discomfort, it often comes with consequences that can impact both your physical and emotional well-being. Consuming high-calorie, low-nutrient comfort foods during emotional episodes can lead to weight gain and poor nutrition. This can create a vicious cycle where weight gain, in turn, triggers more emotional distress, perpetuating the urge to eat emotionally.

Beyond the physical consequences, emotional eating can also take a toll on your emotional health. It can lead to feelings of guilt, shame, and a sense of loss of control. Over time, this can erode self-esteem and further exacerbate emotional issues. Recognizing and addressing emotional eating is essential for breaking this cycle and nurturing a healthier relationship with food and emotions.

In the chapters that follow, we'll explore the intricacies of emotional eating, from the underlying psychological factors to practical strategies for managing it. We'll also delve into the pivotal role of mindset in overcoming emotional eating, which will equip you with the tools needed to navigate this challenging but conquerable aspect of your weight loss journey.

Chapter 2: The Mind-Body Connection

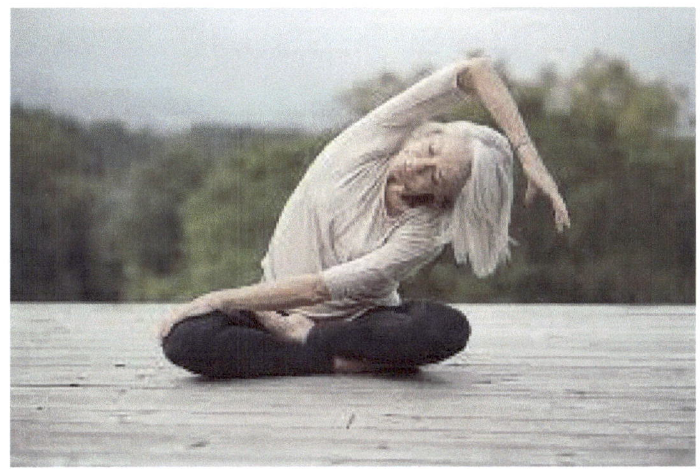

A. Exploring the Mind-Body Connection in Weight Loss

The journey to successful weight loss is more than just numbers on a scale; it's a holistic process that intertwines both the mind and body. Understanding the mind-body connection in weight loss is crucial for achieving sustainable results. The mind and body are not separate entities but are intricately linked, and the choices you make are influenced by your thoughts, emotions, and physical sensations.

Your mindset plays a significant role in your ability to commit to a weight loss plan, stay motivated, and overcome challenges. It affects how you perceive your progress, respond to setbacks, and maintain your long-term goals. Your mental state can either empower you to succeed or hinder your progress. We'll explore how to harness the power of your mind to work in harmony with your body in your weight loss journey.

B. **How Emotions Affect Physical Health**

Emotions are not solely confined to the realm of thoughts and feelings; they have a profound impact on your physical health. When you experience stress, anxiety, or other negative emotions, your body can respond with physiological changes. Stress, for example, triggers the release of hormones like cortisol, which can lead to increased appetite and fat storage, especially around the abdominal area. It can also weaken the immune system and disrupt sleep patterns.

Similarly, emotional eating, often driven by stress or other negative emotions, can lead to unhealthy food choices that negatively impact your physical health. The high consumption of sugary or fatty comfort foods can result in weight gain, elevated blood sugar levels, and an increased risk of chronic health conditions, such as heart disease and diabetes.

Understanding how emotions affect your physical health is essential for creating a comprehensive weight loss strategy. By addressing the emotional aspects of your relationship with food and your mindset, you not only improve your emotional well-being but also positively impact your body's health.

In the chapters that follow, we will explore practical techniques and strategies to strengthen the mind-body connection, enabling you to navigate the complex interplay between emotions, thoughts, and physical health on your path to overcoming emotional eating and achieving your weight loss goals.

Chapter 3: Identifying Your Emotional Triggers

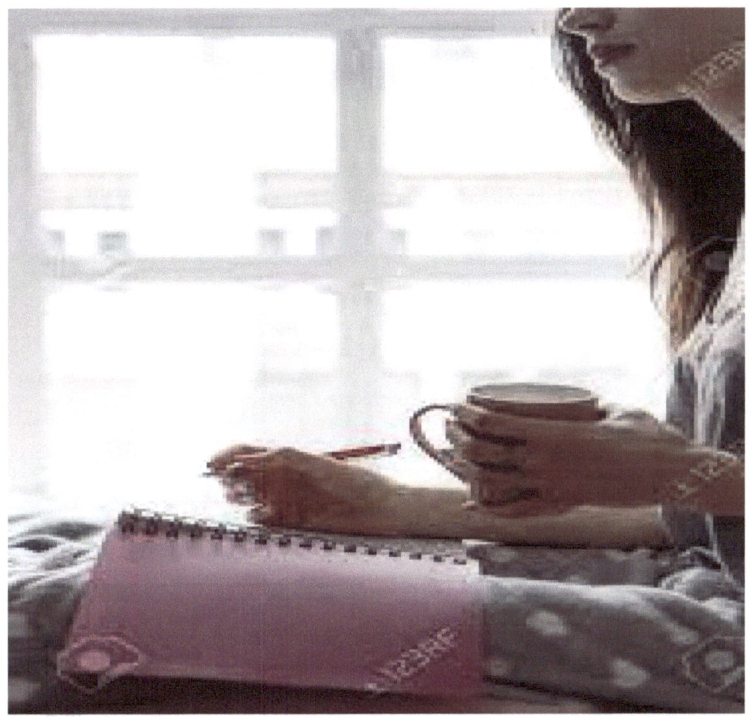

A. Self-assessment Tools and Exercises

To conquer emotional eating and overcome mindset barriers, it's essential to begin by identifying your emotional triggers. Self-assessment tools and exercises can serve as your compass on this introspective journey. They help you gain insight into your emotions, habits, and behaviors. These tools may include questionnaires, quizzes, or guided exercises designed to uncover your emotional relationship with food.

Take the time to honestly evaluate your emotions and the role food plays in your life. Reflect on your eating habits and note instances where you turn to food when you're not physically hungry. Self-assessment tools can provide valuable data for recognizing patterns and triggers that lead to emotional eating.

B. **Recognizing Patterns and Triggers**

Once you've initiated your self-assessment, the next step is to recognize patterns and triggers. Patterns often emerge when you scrutinize your past behaviors. Look for recurring situations, emotions, or events that consistently prompt you to eat emotionally. It could be stress from work, loneliness, arguments, or even celebrations. Identifying these patterns enables you to prepare for potential triggers and implement strategies to manage your emotional responses.

Moreover, it's essential to remember that triggers are not just external events; they can also be internal, stemming from thoughts and self-talk. For instance, negative self-perceptions or beliefs about food can become powerful triggers for emotional eating. As you delve deeper into recognizing these patterns, you'll be better equipped to address them head-on.

C. **Journaling for Self-Awareness**

Journaling is a potent tool for self-awareness and exploration of your relationship with food and emotions. Keeping a journal allows you to document your daily experiences, thoughts, and emotions related to eating. This practice can unveil connections between your mood and eating behaviors that you might have previously overlooked.

When you consistently record your feelings and food choices, you gain insight into your emotional triggers and how they influence your eating patterns. Journaling can serve as a therapeutic outlet for processing your emotions, tracking progress, and developing strategies to overcome emotional eating.

In the upcoming chapters, we will explore strategies and techniques to address and manage these triggers, ultimately breaking free from emotional eating patterns and enhancing your ability to develop a healthier mindset toward food and weight loss. By identifying your emotional triggers, you're taking a significant step towards regaining control over your relationship with food and your emotional well-being.

Chapter 4: Overcoming Mindset Barriers

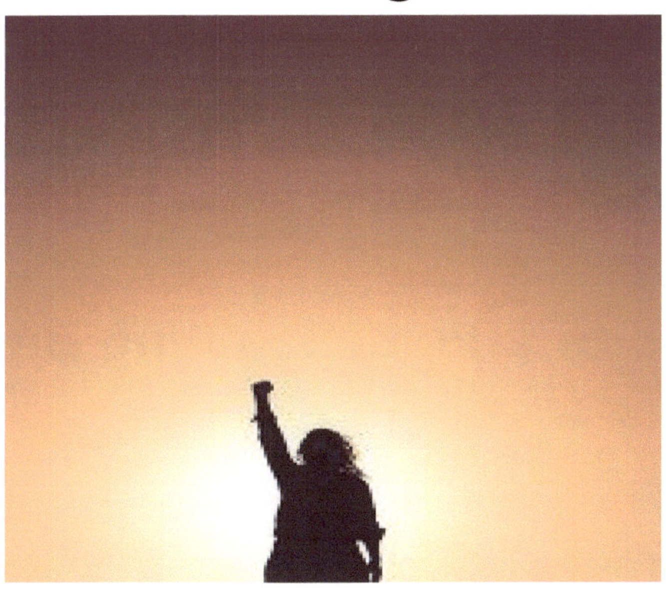

A. Common Mindset Barriers to Weight Loss

As you embark on your journey to conquer emotional eating and achieve your weight loss goals, you'll encounter a series of mindset barriers that can impede your progress. It's vital to recognize these common obstacles that many individuals face when striving for a healthier life. Some of these barriers include self-doubt, fear of failure, negative self-perceptions, and an unhealthy relationship with food.

These mindset barriers often manifest as limiting beliefs that shape your thoughts, emotions, and actions. They can erode your self-esteem and reinforce the cycle of emotional eating. The good news is that by acknowledging these barriers, you can begin to address and overcome them.

B. **Strategies to Change Limiting Beliefs**

Changing limiting beliefs is a fundamental step in overcoming mindset barriers and fostering a positive relationship with food and your body. To challenge and alter these beliefs, you must first identify them. Self-awareness is the key to recognizing the negative thought patterns that hold you back.

Once you've pinpointed your limiting beliefs, you can employ various strategies to challenge and replace them with more constructive and empowering thoughts. Cognitive-behavioral techniques, such as cognitive restructuring, can help you reframe negative beliefs and replace them with positive, growth-oriented affirmations.

Additionally, seeking support from a therapist, counselor, or a support group can be invaluable in addressing deep-seated limiting beliefs. They can guide you through the process of changing your thought patterns and rebuilding your self-image.

C. **Cultivating a Growth Mindset**

A growth mindset is a powerful tool in your journey to overcome emotional eating and achieve sustainable weight loss. This mindset, championed by psychologist Carol Dweck, is the belief that your abilities and intelligence can be developed through dedication and hard work. It stands in stark contrast to a fixed mindset, which believes that abilities are innate and unchangeable.

By cultivating a growth mindset, you view setbacks and challenges as opportunities for growth rather than as failures. It allows you to persevere in the face of adversity, learn from your mistakes, and adapt your strategies. When it comes to emotional eating and weight loss, a growth mindset enables you to embrace the journey as a learning process and to bounce back from setbacks with resilience.

In the chapters ahead, we will delve deeper into practical exercises and strategies to nurture a growth mindset, challenge limiting beliefs, and overcome the mindset barriers that hinder your progress. By reshaping your mindset, you will unlock your full potential in your quest to overcome emotional eating and achieve your weight loss goals.

Chapter 5: Mindful Eating

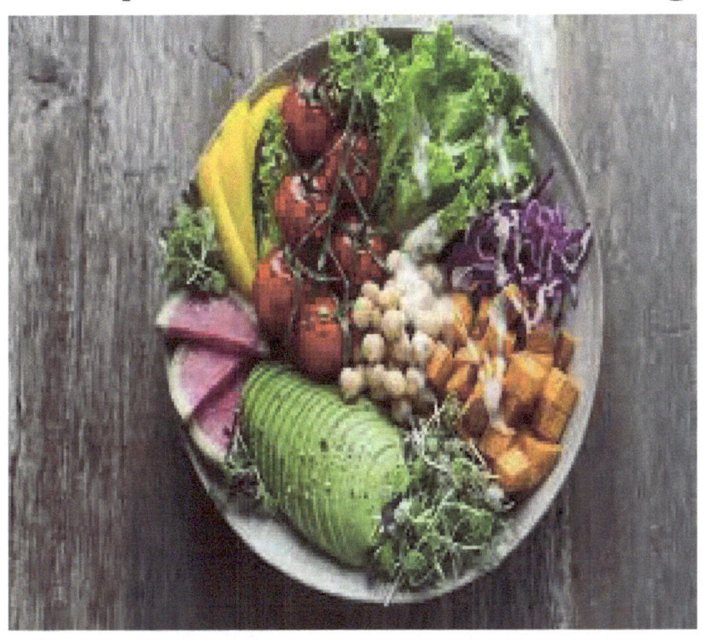

A. Introduction to Mindful Eating

Mindful eating is a powerful practice that can transform your relationship with food and help you overcome emotional eating while enhancing your mindset for weight loss. At its core, mindful eating is about being fully present in the moment during your meals. It's the opposite of mindless or emotional eating, which often involves eating while distracted, stressed, or overwhelmed.

When you eat mindfully, you engage all your senses in the experience of eating. You savor the flavors, textures, and aromas of your food. Mindful eating is not about rigid diets or strict rules. Instead, it's a gentle and non-judgmental approach to nourishing your body and connecting with the experience of eating.

B. **Mindful Eating Techniques and Practices**

There are various techniques and practices you can employ to cultivate mindful eating. These include:

1. **Sensory Awareness**: Pay close attention to the taste, texture, and smell of your food. Let each bite be a sensory experience.

2. **Eating Slowly**: Chew your food slowly and savor each bite. Put your utensils down between mouthfuls to prevent rushing through your meal.

3. **Portion Control**: Be mindful of portion sizes. Serve yourself reasonable amounts and pay attention to your body's hunger and fullness cues.

4. **Eliminating Distractions**: Create a calm eating environment by turning off the TV, putting away your phone, and sitting at a table.

5. **Emotional Check-In**: Before you eat, take a moment to check in with your emotions. Are you eating out of hunger, boredom, stress, or genuine enjoyment of the food?

6. **Expressing Gratitude**: Express gratitude for the food on your plate and the nourishment it provides to your body.

C. **Benefits of Mindful Eating**

Mindful eating offers a multitude of benefits, particularly in the context of overcoming emotional eating and achieving sustainable weight loss. Some of these benefits include:

1. **Improved Awareness**: Mindful eating increases your awareness of your eating habits

and emotional triggers, helping you make conscious choices.

2. **Weight Management**: By eating more slowly and savoring your food, you are more likely to recognize when you're full, making it easier to control portion sizes and maintain a healthy weight.

3. **Emotion Regulation**: Mindful eating helps you become more attuned to your emotions and enables you to respond to them in healthier ways than turning to food.

4. **Enhanced Digestion**: Eating mindfully aids in better digestion as you give your body the time it needs to process food efficiently.

5. **Reduced Stress**: The practice of mindfulness during meals can reduce stress levels and promote a sense of calm and well-being.

In the chapters that follow, we will delve deeper into the art of mindful eating, providing you with practical exercises and guidance to incorporate this transformative practice into your daily life. By embracing mindful eating, you'll not only gain better control over your relationship with food but also harness the power of mindfulness to enhance your mindset for successful weight loss.

Chapter 6: Building a Support System

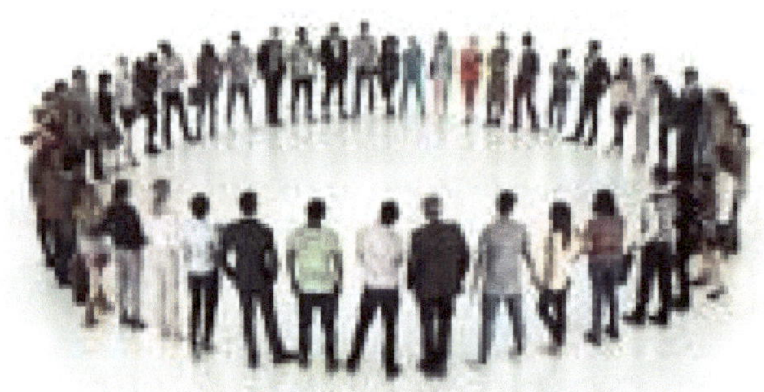

A. **The Importance of a Support System**

When it comes to embarking on a journey of emotional eating recovery and weight loss, a robust support system can be a game-changer. The path may be challenging at times, and having a network of individuals who understand and encourage your goals can provide invaluable assistance. A support system offers several key advantages:

1. **Accountability**: Knowing that someone is there to support and check in on your progress can help keep you accountable to your goals.

2. **Emotional Support**: Dealing with emotional eating and weight loss can be emotionally taxing. Having people who understand and offer emotional support can help you cope with the ups and downs.

3. **Motivation**: A strong support system can provide the motivation and inspiration you need to stay committed to your journey.

4. **Shared Resources**: Your support system can offer advice, tips, and resources that you might not have discovered on your own.

B. Finding Support in Your Community

Support can come from a variety of sources within your local community. Here are a few places to consider when building your support system:

1. **Friends and Family**: Often, the most immediate support network is your friends and

family. Share your goals with them and seek their understanding and encouragement.

2. **Local Support Groups**: Many communities have support groups for individuals dealing with emotional eating and weight loss. These groups provide a safe space to share experiences and strategies.

3. **Therapists and Counselors:** Professional support is invaluable. Consider working with a therapist or counselor who specializes in emotional eating and weight management.

4. **Fitness Classes or Clubs**: Joining local fitness classes or clubs can connect you with like-minded individuals who are on their own health and wellness journey.

C. Online Resources and Communities

The digital age has opened up a wealth of online resources and communities dedicated to emotional eating and weight loss support. Here's how you can tap into this vast network:

1. **Online Forums and Groups**: Many websites and social media platforms host forums and groups focused on emotional eating and weight loss. These can be excellent places to share your experiences, seek advice, and offer support to others.

2. **Apps and Online Tools**: There are numerous apps and online tools designed to help you track your progress, set goals, and connect with others who share your journey.

3. **Virtual Coaching**: Consider virtual coaching or counseling sessions if you prefer one-on-one support without leaving your home.

4. **Blogs and Podcasts**: Numerous bloggers and podcasters share their personal journeys and expert advice on emotional eating and weight

loss. These can provide valuable insights and inspiration.

In the upcoming chapters, we will continue to explore strategies and practices to strengthen your support system, providing you with the guidance you need to maintain your commitment to overcoming emotional eating and achieving your weight loss goals. Your support system, whether local or virtual, will play a crucial role in your success.

Chapter 7: Creating a Sustainable Weight Loss Plan

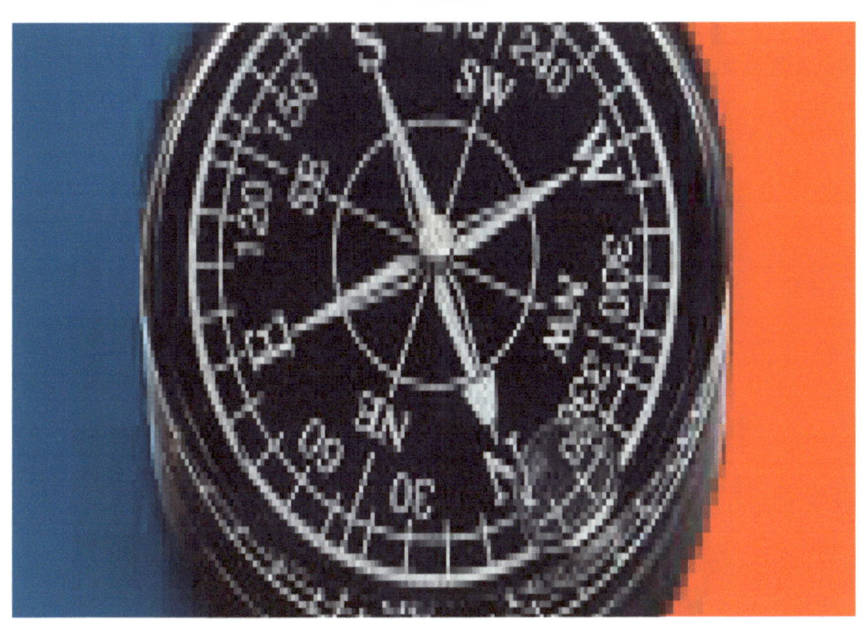

A. Setting Realistic Goals

When it comes to weight loss, setting realistic goals is a cornerstone of success. Your goals should be achievable and tailored to your unique circumstances. Here's how to set realistic weight loss goals:

1. **Be Specific**: Clearly define your goals. Instead of saying "I want to lose weight," specify how much weight you aim to lose and by when.

2. **Break It Down**: Divide your larger goal into smaller, more achievable milestones. This makes the process more manageable and less overwhelming.

3. **Consider Time**: Give yourself a realistic timeframe for achieving your goals. Remember that slow, steady progress is often more sustainable than rapid weight loss.

4. **Account for Lifestyle**: Your goals should align with your lifestyle. Don't set objectives that require radical changes that you can't sustain in the long run.

B. Designing a Personalized Weight Loss Plan

A one-size-fits-all approach to weight loss often falls short in addressing emotional eating and mindset barriers. Designing a personalized plan tailored to your specific needs and preferences is vital. Here's how to create such a plan:

1. **Assessment**: Evaluate your current habits, preferences, and obstacles. Understand what drives your emotional eating and what strategies have worked for you in the past.

2. **Set Clear Objectives**: Based on your assessment, define clear and specific objectives that address both emotional eating triggers and weight loss goals.

3. **Nutrition Plan**: Create a balanced nutrition plan that aligns with your goals. Ensure it includes a variety of foods that you enjoy and that provide essential nutrients.

4. **Exercise Routine**: Incorporate physical activity that you enjoy and can commit to. Find ways to make exercise a part of your routine, even if it's just a daily walk.

5. **Behavioral Strategies**: Implement strategies to address emotional eating, such as mindfulness

techniques and coping mechanisms for dealing with emotional triggers.

C. **Incorporating Long-Term Strategies**

Sustainable weight loss is not just about shedding pounds; it's about maintaining a healthy lifestyle for the long term. Consider these strategies for the journey ahead:

1. **Lifestyle Changes**: Focus on adopting healthy lifestyle changes that you can maintain even after reaching your weight loss goals.

2. **Consistency**: Consistency is key. Stick to your plan and adapt it as needed to ensure long-term success.

3. **Mindfulness**: Continue to practice mindful eating to stay in tune with your body's hunger and fullness cues.

4. **Regular Check-Ins**: Periodically reassess your goals and progress. Adjust your plan as necessary to accommodate changes in your life.

5. **Support System**: Leverage your support system to stay motivated and accountable as you work toward maintaining your healthier lifestyle.

In the chapters that follow, we'll dive deeper into these aspects of creating a sustainable weight loss plan. By setting realistic goals, designing a personalized plan, and incorporating long-term strategies, you'll be well-prepared to overcome emotional eating, develop a healthier mindset, and achieve lasting success on your weight loss journey.

Chapter 8: Coping with Setbacks

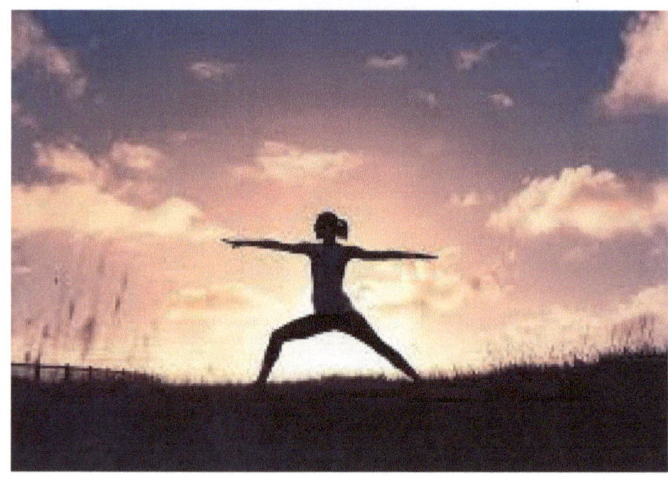

A. How to Handle Relapses and Setbacks

Setbacks and relapses are a natural part of the journey toward overcoming emotional eating and achieving your weight loss goals. It's essential to recognize that encountering challenges doesn't equate to failure. Instead, they provide opportunities for learning and growth. Here's how to effectively handle relapses and setbacks:

1. **Self-Compassion**: Be kind and understanding to yourself. Understand that everyone faces setbacks, and they don't define your worth or potential for success.

2. **Reflect and Learn**: Instead of dwelling on the setback, use it as an opportunity to reflect and learn. What triggered the emotional eating episode? What could you have done differently?

3. **Revisit Your Goals**: Reevaluate your goals and assess whether they are realistic and sustainable. Adjust them as necessary based on what you've learned.

4. **Seek Support**: Reach out to your support system for guidance and encouragement. They can help you regain perspective and motivation.

5. **Mindfulness**: Use mindfulness techniques to navigate the emotional aftermath of setbacks. Be aware of your emotions, acknowledge them, and choose healthier ways to cope.

B. Developing Resilience and Self-Compassion

Developing resilience and self-compassion is crucial for long-term success. These qualities will help you bounce back from setbacks and continue your journey with determination. Here's how to cultivate resilience and self-compassion:

1. **Accept Imperfection**: Understand that perfection is not the goal. Accept that setbacks are part of the process, and they don't diminish your progress.

2. **Positive Self-Talk**: Replace negative self-talk with positive affirmations. Encourage yourself, and remember that you are capable of overcoming challenges.

3. **Resilience Training**: Develop resilience through practices like stress management, problem-solving, and seeking constructive solutions.

4. **Supportive Network**: Surround yourself with a supportive network that reminds you of your worth and encourages self-compassion.

5. **Mindfulness and Self-Car**e: Engage in mindfulness practices and self-care routines that nourish your emotional well-being. This includes activities that help you relax, de-stress, and find balance.

As you move forward on your journey to overcome emotional eating and achieve your weight loss goals, remember that setbacks do not define your path. Instead, they serve as opportunities to refine your approach, develop resilience, and practice self-compassion. By embracing these qualities, you'll be better equipped to navigate the challenges and uncertainties that arise along the way, ultimately strengthening your mindset and increasing your likelihood of long-term success.

Conclusion

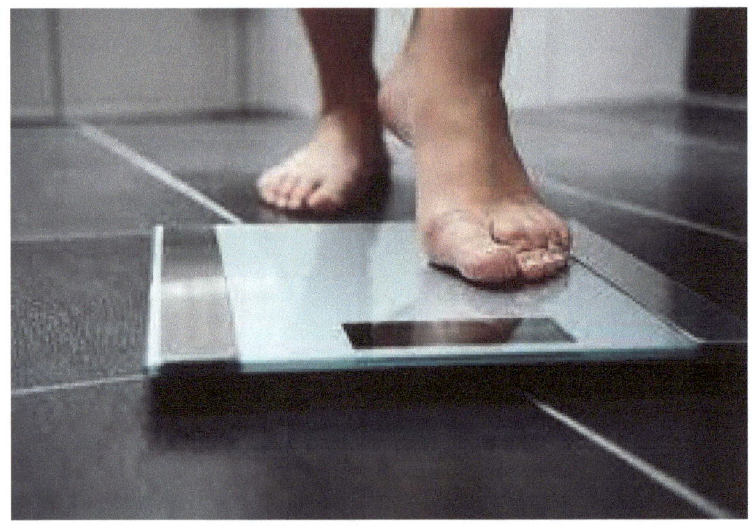

A. **Summarizing Key Takeaways**

In the pages of "Emotional Eating Uncovered: Overcoming Mindset Barriers for Weight Loss," we've embarked on a transformative journey to understand the intricate relationship between emotions and eating, and how your mindset plays a pivotal role in your quest for weight loss. Let's recap the key takeaways from this exploration:

- **Emotional Eating**: We've unraveled the concept of emotional eating, understanding that it's not a sign of weakness but a common response to emotions. Recognizing and addressing emotional eating is the first step towards lasting change.

- **Mind-Body Connection**: We've explored the profound connection between your mind and body in the weight loss process. By acknowledging this connection, you can harness the power of your mindset for positive change.

- **Identifying Triggers**: Chapter 3 guided you in identifying your emotional triggers, using self-assessment tools, recognizing patterns, and practicing journaling for self-awareness.

- **Overcoming Mindset Barriers**: In Chapter 4, we discovered common mindset barriers and how to challenge them, emphasizing the importance of cultivating a growth mindset.

- **Mindful Eating**: Chapter 5 introduced you to the art of mindful eating, offering techniques and practices to help you savor your food and be present during meals.

- **Building a Support System**: We learned the significance of a support system in Chapter 6, with a focus on finding support in your local community and online resources.

- **Creating a Sustainable Weight Loss Plan**: Chapter 7 emphasized the importance of setting realistic goals, designing a personalized weight loss plan, and incorporating long-term strategies.

- **Coping with Setbacks**: In Chapter 8, we discussed how to handle relapses and setbacks, highlighting the importance of self-compassion and resilience.

B. Encouragement for the Journey Ahead

As you close this book and prepare to continue your journey, remember that you possess the knowledge, tools, and resilience needed to overcome emotional eating and achieve your weight loss goals. You are not alone on this path. Your support system, whether it's family, friends, support groups, or online communities, is there to bolster your efforts.

The road ahead may present challenges, but it's through these challenges that we grow and discover our true potential. Be patient with yourself, and embrace self-compassion in moments of difficulty. Know that setbacks are not failures but stepping stones towards progress.

Your journey to overcoming emotional eating and fostering a healthier mindset is a testament to your commitment to a better, healthier, and more balanced life. You have the strength to transform your relationship with food and emotions, achieving the weight loss goals that matter to you.

Keep the knowledge you've gained within these pages close to your heart, and may it guide you through the ups and downs of this transformative journey. Your story is unique, and your success is within reach. With determination, self-compassion, and a positive mindset, you can uncover the healthier, happier you that awaits on the other side of emotional eating.

You've got this. Your journey continues, and the best is yet to come.

www.ingramcontent.com/pod-product-compliance
Lightning Source LLC
Chambersburg PA
CBHW040050240726
48664CB00004B/1131